HANDBOOK OF PRESCHOOL MENTAL HEALTH

HANDBOOK OF PRESCHOOL MENTAL HEALTH
Development, Disorders, and Treatment

Edited by
JOAN L. LUBY

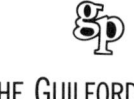

THE GUILFORD PRESS
New York   London

© 2006 The Guilford Press
A Division of Guilford Publications, Inc.
72 Spring Street, New York, NY 10012
www.guilford.com

Printed in the United States of America

This book is printed on acid-free paper.

Last digit is print number: 9 8 7 6 5 4 3 2 1

Library of Congress Cataloging-in-Publication Data

Handbook of preschool mental health : development, disorders, and treatment /
  edited by Joan L. Luby.
       p. ; cm.
  Includes bibliographical references and index.
  ISBN-13: 978-1-59385-313-6 (alk. paper)
  ISBN-10: 1-59385-313-0 (alk. paper)
  1. Child psychiatry—Handbooks, manuals, etc. 2. Preschool children—
Mental health—Handbooks, manuals, etc.
  [DNLM: 1. Mental Disorders—physiopathology. 2. Child Development.
3. Child Psychology. 4. Child, Preschool. 5. Mental Disorders—therapy.
WS 350 H23597 2006] I. Luby, Joan L.
  RJ499.H36 2006
  618.92′89—dc22

                                                              2006000352

"For Warmth" reprinted from *Call Me by My True Name* (1999) by Thich Nhat Hanh
with permission of Parallax Press, Berkeley, California, www.parallax.org.

To my parents, Elliot and Ideane Luby,
who, with tremendous love and generosity,
helped me to realize my intellectual dreams

About the Editor

Joan L. Luby, MD, is an infant/preschool psychiatrist and Associate Professor of Child Psychiatry at the Washington University School of Medicine in St. Louis, where she is the founder and director of the Early Emotional Development Program. This clinical and research program focusing on mood disorders in preschool children was the first of its kind nationally. Dr. Luby has been awarded grants from the National Institute of Mental Heath and the National Alliance for Schizophrenia and Depression, which have supported her research on the phenomenology of early-onset mood disorders. She currently chairs the Infancy Committee of the American Academy of Child and Adolescent Psychiatry and serves on several scientific advisory groups focused on the development of age-appropriate diagnostic criteria for preschool disorders.

Contributors

Thomas F. Anders, MD, Department of Psychiatry and Behavioral Sciences, University of California, Davis, M.I.N.D. Institute, Sacramento, California

Adrian Angold, MRCPsych, Center for Developmental Epidemiology, Department of Psychiatry and Behavioral Sciences, Duke University Medical Center, Durham, North Carolina

Andy C. Belden, PhD, Department of Child Psychiatry, Washington University School of Medicine, St. Louis, Missouri

Anne Leland Benham, PhD, Department of Psychiatry and Behavioral Sciences, Stanford University School of Medicine, Palo Alto, California

Somer L. Bishop, MA, Department of Psychology, University of Michigan, Ann Arbor, Michigan

Melissa M. Burnham, PhD, Department of Human Development and Family Studies, University of Nevada, Reno, Reno, Nevada

Irene Chatoor, MD, Department of Psychiatry and Pediatrics, George Washington University, and Children's National Medical Center, Washington, DC

Brent R. Collett, PhD, Department of Psychiatry and Behavioral Sciences, University of Washington School of Medicine, and Children's Hospital and Regional Medical Center, Seattle, Washington

Geraldine Dawson, PhD, Department of Psychology and University of Washington Autism Center, University of Washington, Seattle, Washington

Susanne A. Denham, PhD, Department of Psychology, George Mason University, Fairfax, Virginia

Helen Link Egger, MD, Center for Developmental Epidemiology and Department of Psychiatry and Behavioral Sciences, Duke University Medical Center, Durham, North Carolina

Susan Faja, MS, Center on Human Development and Disabilities, University of Washington, Seattle, Washington

Erika E. Gaylor, PhD, Center for Education and Human Services, Policy Division, SRI International, Menlo Park, California

Rebecca Goodvin, MA, Department of Psychology, University of Nebraska, Lincoln, Nebraska

Amy K. Heffelfinger, PhD, Departments of Neurology and Neurosurgery, Medical College of Wisconsin, Milwaukee, Wisconsin

Audrey Kapilinsky, LCSW, Child Development Center, University of California, Irvine, Irvine, California

Deepa Khushlani, MD, Department of Psychiatry and Behavioral Medicine, Children's National Medical Center, Washington, DC

Ron Kotkin, PhD, Department of Pediatrics and Child Development Center, University of California, Irvine, Irvine, California

Marc Lerner, MD, Department of Pediatrics, University of California, Irvine, Irvine, California

Alicia F. Lieberman, PhD, Department of Psychiatry, University of California, San Francisco, San Francisco, California

Catherine Lord, PhD, Department of Psychology and Psychiatry, University of Michigan Autism and Communication Disorders Center, Ann Arbor, Michigan

Joan L. Luby, MD, Department of Psychiatry, Washington University School of Medicine, St. Louis, Missouri

Jon M. McClellan, MD, Department of Psychiatry and Behavioral Sciences, University of Washington School of Medicine, and Children's Hospital and Regional Medical Center, Seattle, Washington

Sara Meyer, MA, Department of Psychology, University of California, Davis, Davis, California

Christine Mrakotsky, PhD, Department of Psychiatry, Harvard Medical School, and Children's Hospital Boston, Boston, Massachusetts

Carol M. Rockhill, MD, PhD, Department of Psychiatry and Behavioral Sciences, University of Washington School of Medicine, Seattle, Washington

Michael S. Scheeringa, MD, MPH, Institute of Infant and Early Childhood Mental Health and Department of Psychiatry and Neurology, Tulane University School of Medicine, New Orleans, Louisiana

Carol Fisher Slotnick, MSW, PhD, Department of Psychiatry and Behavioral Sciences, Stanford University School of Medicine, Palo Alto, California

Matthew L. Speltz, PhD, Department of Psychiatry and Behavioral Sciences, University of Washington School of Medicine, and Children's Hospital and Regional Medical Center, Seattle, Washington

Brian S. Stafford, MD, MPH, Department of Pediatrics and Child Psychology, Denver Children's Hospital, and The Kempe Center, Denver, Colorado

Robin Steinberg-Epstein, MD, Department of Pediatrics, University of California, Irvine, Irvine, California

Kenneth W. Steinhoff, MD, UCI Child Development Center, University of California, Irvine, Irvine, California

James M. Swanson, PhD, UCI Child Development Center, University of California, Irvine, Irvine, California

Ross A. Thompson, PhD, Department of Psychology, University of California, Davis, Davis, California

Patricia Van Horn, PhD, Department of Psychiatry, University of California, San Francisco, San Francisco, California

Sharon Wigal, PhD, Department of Pediatrics, University of California, Irvine, Irvine, California

Tim Wigal, PhD, Department of Pediatrics, University of California, Irvine, Irvine, California

Charles H. Zeanah, MD, Department of Psychiatry and Pediatrics, Tulane University, New Orleans, Louisiana

Preface

For Warmth
I hold my face between my hands
    no I am not crying
I hold my face between my hands
    to keep my loneliness warm
      two hands protecting
      two hands nourishing
      two hands to prevent
my soul from leaving me
      in anger.
        —THICH NHAT HANH

In so few words, this poem beautifully captures what is so vital about early emotional development and its importance in the human condition. It is the willingness and ability to embrace fully and experience the broad spectrum of emotional states, including those that are painful and distressing, that may be key to mental health and adaptive personal development. As psychoanalytic theory has suggested for decades, by achieving this emotional developmental capacity, one gains the ability to have a clear view of oneself and others, and to engage fully and honestly in the human experience and all of its vicissitudes. Guiding young children's development in this area early in life could be as empowering as learning to walk or talk. However, because of its intangible quality and our own limited mastery of this as adults, this goal has eluded us thus far.

This volume aims to discuss early-onset mental disorders in preschool-age children from a fundamentally developmental perspective. To achieve this goal, the first section of the book is devoted to a review of the available empirical developmental literature pertaining to those areas that have a direct relevance to mental disorders. This includes a review of new data on the development of self-concept (Chapter 1), emotions and socialization (Chapter 2), and cognition (Chapter 3). There are surprising gaps in the developmental literature on many basic elements of the development of emotions, although key elements of the available literature in this area are reviewed in Chapter 10 on mood disorders as they pertain to our understanding of normative and aberrant affect early in life.

Although child mental health providers would agree in principle that a fundamental knowledge of normative development is essential to practice, this is often given short shrift in training and in clinical application. When developmental principles are applied, they tend to be anecdotal, informal, and therefore inexact. As we attempt to identify mental disorders in younger and younger populations, a more detailed knowledge of these elements becomes essential as we aim to differentiate clinically significant problems from the normative and transient emotional and behavioral extremes and difficulties of early development.

Over the last decade, significant progress has been made in the understanding of mental disorders in preschoolers, who range in age from 3 to 6 years, while much has been known about children older than 6 for some time. Part II provides a comprehensive review of the available empirical findings for each diagnostic category in which a substantial body of data was found. Chapters 6 and 9 on eating and sleeping disorders, respectively, give an up-to-date and clinically pragmatic account of how these problems that cross the clinical threshold present in the preschool period. Chapters 7 and 10 on anxiety and mood disorders, respectively, as well as Chapter 8 on posttraumatic stress disorder (PTSD), review the empirical database. Work on mood disorders and PTSD has achieved considerable momentum in the area of validation and clarification of age-adjusted symptoms.

There is a substantial body of work on the identification of autism spectrum disorders in the preschool period, which is the latest developmental period that one should aim to capture these disorders. New empirical findings have emerged on preschool attention-deficit/hyperactivity disorder from a multisite treatment study (see Chapter 4). These findings are useful to inform both diagnosis and treatment. These chapters are designed to be of use to clinicians of all disciplines as a source of information on how to diagnose properly and begin to formulate treatment strategies for very-early-onset disorders.

Although the area of specific treatments for preschool disorders remains a largely empirically unexplored area, the chapters contained in Part III review the state of our knowledge of treatment modalities specifically designed for preschoolers. Areas covered range from dyadic play therapies (Chapters 15 and 16) to psychopharmacology (Chapter 14). Chapters focus on the theoretical (e.g., play therapy) to highly empirical (e.g., treatment of autism spectrum disorders; Chapter 17), varying with the available data base specific to each diagnostic area.

Chapter 14 on psychopharmacology broadly reviews the scant available empirical studies as they apply to the range of conditions identified and treated in young children. Given the substantial gaps in the literature, the chapter outlines recommendations for future research. Basic guidelines and principles for the prescribing physician are also offered to help inform clinical decision making in this area in which there is substantial social pressure on the physician to prescribe in the absence of empirical data to guide these treatment decisions. Part III also includes Chapter 13 on neuropsychological assessment of preschool-age children. This is a developing area, with new, age-specific assessment methods that may serve as a useful adjunct to a diagnostic assessment.

Whereas the chapters presented in this volume are of obvious use to clinicians and researchers who focus on young children, the principles outlined may also be useful and applicable for practitioners who assess and treat mental disorders across the lifespan. In particular, the developmental perspective can be used to formulate more informed hypotheses about etiologies and may also be surprisingly useful to assess adaptive functioning in individuals across the age range. In this way, they may also be applicable to prevention and personal growth models.

The Buddhist spiritual leader and author Thich Nhat Hanh, and others like him, serve as a model for individuals seeking greater emotional sentience, as well as for those seeking relief from emotional suffering. I am grateful and humbled by my own experiences of suffering, which I continue to try "to keep warm." As his gracefully crafted words convey, the practice of fully experiencing and simultaneously regulating a broad array of appropriate emotions is important, because it enhances one's ability to experience joy in all its intensity, as joy emerges from anguish (as one example), and in this way to participate fully in and enjoy human relationships. These principles have also helped me to have a clearer view of emotions, their range and repertoire, and to apply this view to my own area of interest, early-onset mood disorders. I believe it is important to keep our loneliness "warm"—as Thich Nhat Hanh suggests, to stay in touch with but not become overwhelmed by loneliness and emotions like it—for balance and understanding to help us identify, tolerate, experience, and modulate these emotions in our children and ourselves.

I hope that this book will be useful to clinicians, developmentalists, and researchers interested in young children. The field of preschool mental health has made substantial progress as advances in our understanding of early development have emerged. The greater awareness of the emotional and cognitive capacities of the young child has opened the door for clinicians and researchers to design age-appropriate approaches to tap internal emotional states in preverbal children. Subsequent findings reviewed in this volume, demonstrating an even earlier onset of many mental disorders than previously recognized, hold promise for investigations of early and potentially more effective intervention. Whereas such advances are welcome news for preschool children, and alone would likely gratify those of us committed to that population, they may also hold promise for impacting the trajectory of mental disorders across the lifespan. It is tremendously exciting and gratifying that the field of preschool mental health has made sufficient progress to fill an edited volume of this size.

Contents

Part III. Assessment and Intervention in the Preschool Period

Part I

Normative Development in the Preschool Period

1

Social Development
Psychological Understanding, Self-Understanding, and Relationships

ROSS A. THOMPSON, REBECCA GOODVIN, and SARA MEYER

All preschoolers are developing individuals. Whether or not they are challenged by autism, anxiety, mood disorders, or other problems of mental health, they are acquiring new forms of self-awareness and social understanding, are striving to understand and manage their emotions, and their psychological development is profoundly influenced by their close relationships with caregivers. The view that typical and atypical children alike face comparable developmental challenges and opportunities is central to the developmental psychopathology perspective that is incorporated into this volume, and has guided theory and research concerning early childhood mental health for the past quarter-century (see Cicchetti & Cohen, 2005). Such a view integrates the special concerns of early mental health problems with the broader challenges of typical development during the preschool years. This integrated view is especially important in light of the pioneering new advances in the conceptualization, prevention, and treatment of early mental health problems in infants and young children. Understanding the developmental processes and influences that shape early social, emotional, and personality development contributes to improved knowledge of the sources of vulnerability and support that can inform the study of preschool mental health.

This chapter, and Chapter 2 by Denham, provides a survey of normative processes of emotional, social, and personality development (see Thompson, 2006, for a more extended discussion of these topics). Here we focus on three facets of early psychological growth that are especially prominent in the preschool years. First, young children dramatically advance in their comprehension of other people and the intentions, desires, emotions, and beliefs that cause people to act as they do, and we summarize these accomplishments in psychological understanding. These achievements are important to mental health because individual differences in social and emotional understanding are associated with social competence, and lack of social competence is a key feature of some psychological disorders. Second, early childhood is a time of equally dramatic advances in self-understanding as young children begin to represent themselves and their characteristics in psychologically relevant ways, and we describe these accomplishments in the next section. Finally, because young children's experiences in close relationships are central to these and other facets of psychological growth, we consider the nature of these relationships and their developmental importance in the third section. Throughout this chapter we consider the mental health implications of these developmental processes and the influences on them.

DEVELOPMENT OF PSYCHOLOGICAL UNDERSTANDING

The traditional view is that young children are egocentric, limited in their comprehension of others' feelings, desires, and thoughts by their cognitive preoccupation with their own viewpoint. Contemporary developmental scientists are, by contrast, amazed by how early and successfully the young child begins to grasp the mental states of other people, even when those emotions, beliefs, and desires are different from the child's own. Young children may sometimes seem egocentric because of their limited social knowledge, such as when they are judging what would be a desirable snack or gift for an adult. But closer examination (using more incisive research methods) has shown that even infants begin to comprehend that subjective mental states are the key to understanding people's behavior, and during the preschool years children acquire a surprisingly sophisticated understanding of the nature of those mental states. The hallmark of psychological understanding during the preschool years is children's developing "theory of mind," which consists of (1) the realization that mental states underlie actions, (2) the diverse sources of those mental states, (3) the realization that mental states are associated with other mental states, and (4) that mental representations of the world may not always be consistent with the reality they represent. These conceptual accomplishments are important, because the capacity to understand the feelings, desires, and thoughts that govern behavior contributes to other essential skills, such as social competence, emotion sensitivity, and a dawning psychological understanding of self.

Infancy: Social Catalysts to Dawning Psychological Understanding

The earliest origins of developing theory of mind begin in infancy, as babies first become intrigued by the social partners surrounding them and seek to discern predictable regularities in their behavior. During episodes of face-to-face play in the early months after birth, for example, infants and their caregivers engage each other in close proximity while interacting with facial expressions, vocalizations, touching, behavioral gestures, and in other ways (Malatesta, Culver, Tesman, & Shepard, 1989; Tronick, 1989). These brief but ubiquitous episodes of focused social interaction have no agenda other than mutual entertainment, but they also provide an early forum for the development of social skills and the growth of the baby's social expectations for the adult. From these exchanges, infants gradually learn that people respond to their initiatives in ways that create excitement; that social interaction is dynamic and changing; and that facial, vocal, and behavioral expressions of emotion go together. Furthermore, because episodes of face-to-face play shift frequently between periods of well-synchronized behavioral coordination and periods of dyssynchrony, infants also learn how their actions and feelings can influence the continuing course of social interaction with a partner (Thompson, 2006).

The importance of this learning can be seen in studies of the "still face" effect in young infants, in which mothers alternate episodes of face-to-face interaction with an episode in which they look at the baby but are impassive and unresponsive. During these intervening perturbation episodes, infants reliably respond with diminished positive affect, withdrawal, self-directed behavior, and sometimes with social elicitations (e.g., brief smiles, momentarily increased vocalizing and reaching) alternating with negative affect. These responses seem to reflect their expectation that the adult should continue to interact animatedly with them. When mothers subsequently respond normally, infants become more sociable but also remain subdued (see Adamson & Frick, 2003, for a review of this literature). Studies have revealed that depressed mothers are less responsive and emotionally more subdued and negative in face-to-face play than are nondepressed mothers, and the offspring of depressed mothers are themselves less responsive and emotionally animated than are typical infants as early as 2–3 months of age (e.g., Cohn, Campbell, Matias, & Hopkins, 1990; Field et al., 1988). Moreover, if maternal depression persists, by the end of the first year, infants exhibit atypical patterns of frontal brain activity related to emotion that are also evident in interaction with other, nondepressed partners (Dawson et al., 1999). Differences in early social responsiveness therefore seem to be important for the development of social expectations and social skills, which may be particularly important for mental health if these capacities develop atypically owing to difficult early relational experiences.

Later in the first year, infants become capable of moving about on their own, and this locomotor accomplishment is accompanied by greater goal directedness and intentionality as babies become capable of approaching objects and people that interest them. This achievement is also accompanied by greater parental monitoring and intervention and, perhaps inevitably, conflicts of will between the infant and protective parents when the infant approaches dangerous or forbidden objects. These conflicts may be conceptually important, however, because they expose infants to social encounters that underscore how others' intentions differ from those of the self (Campos et al., 1999). Perhaps because of experiences like these, elegant experimental studies by Woodward and others have shown that by 9–12 months infants begin to perceive other people as intentional, goal-oriented actors (see Woodward, Sommerville, & Guajardo, 2001). It appears, in other words, that when watching other people reaching, pointing, or acting in an object-oriented way, infants begin to perceive those actions as goal-directed. They are assisted in this realization by sensitive caregivers who are themselves attuned to the intentional orientation of behavior, and who often punctuate their verbal responses to their own goal-oriented activity, or to the infant's goal-directed efforts, with affirmative utterances whenever the goal has been accomplished.

By the end of the first year, therefore, infants have begun to perceive other people as subjective, intentional agents whose goals may or may not be the same as the infant's own. They show this awareness in many ways, such as in the creation of joint attentional states with adults, and in social referencing behavior. Infants create joint attention with adults when they look in the direction of the adult's gaze or look from an object to the adult's face and back to the object again. Such initiatives reflect a rudimentary awareness of the association between attentional direction and subjective focus, and sometimes also seem intended to alter the adult's subjective orientation to elicit a desired response (e.g., getting access to the object, such as a toy, by redirecting the adult's attention to it; see Tomasello & Rakoczy, 2003). "Social referencing" occurs when a person uses another's emotional cues to interpret an uncertain event, and can be observed when 1-year-olds scan the mother's face in an unfamiliar situation (Baldwin & Moses, 1996). Such events show that by the end of the first year, infants are good consumers of emotional cues, and they are acquiring an understanding that others' emotions can be evoked by specific objects or events that the infant also sees, and infants can use this understanding to guide their own interpretation of that event. Taken together, research on joint attention and social referencing portrays the 1-year-old as having a surprisingly nonegocentric regard for people as intentional agents with subjective viewpoints that can, at times, be monitored and altered.

Understanding People's Desires and Emotions

Toddlers expand their developing theory of mind as they comprehend how people's actions are guided by their desires and emotions. These psychological states are actually quite challenging for young children to comprehend, because they are invisible, multidetermined motivators of behavior. But as early as 18 months, children already exhibit a rudimentary comprehension of the importance of differences in desire. In one study, Repacholi and Gopnik (1997) presented 14- and 18-month-olds with two snacks: goldfish crackers (the children's favorite) and broccoli (which the children disliked). Then the adult tasted each snack, smiling and exhibiting pleasure ("Mmmm!") with one, and frowning and saying "Ewwww!" with the other. In the "match" condition, the adult's preferences were the same as the child's; in the "mismatch" condition, the adult preferred the broccoli and disliked the crackers. Then the adult extended her hand and said, "I want some more; can you give me more?" The 18-month-olds reliably gave the adult the food she desired in both the match and mismatch conditions. By contrast, the 14-month-olds overwhelmingly gave the adult more goldfish crackers in each condition. The sensitivity to differences in desire among 18-month-olds (especially when the adult's desire contrasted with the child's own preferences) is consistent with evidence that spontaneous verbal references to desire emerge by 18 months, and that somewhat later children begin to offer constrastive statements about desire, such as comparing what one person wants with what another desires (Bartsch & Wellman, 1995).

By age 2, toddlers also begin spontaneously to talk about emotions, the causes of emotions, and even emotional regulatory efforts (e.g., Bartsch & Wellman, 1995; Wellman, Harris, Banerjee, & Sinclair, 1995). Careful analyses of the content of these utterances show that children of this age regard emotions as subjective, psychological conditions that can vary between people, with young children often contrasting another's emotions with their own. Later in the third year, toddlers comprehend the connections between desires and emotions (e.g., people are happy when they get what they want, and unhappy when they do not) (Wellman & Woolley, 1990). By age 3, children have begun to understand how emotions are associated with beliefs and expectations about events, such as the surprise a visitor feels after seeing giraffes on a farm (Wellman & Banerjee, 1991). Young children's comprehension of the connection between emotion and thought is also revealed in their appreciation of how feelings can be evoked by mental reminders of past emotionally evocative experiences. By age 5, for example, children understand that someone can feel sad when seeing a cat that reminds her of a pet who ran away (Lagattuta & Wellman, 2001). These insights not only help young children comprehend the origins and consequences of others' feelings but also contribute to children's understanding of their own emotions and how to manage them (Thompson, 1994).

Comprehending Beliefs—and False Beliefs

Consider the following situation: An experimenter shows a child a candy box and asks the child what she thinks is inside. The child replies, naturally, "Candy!" The box is opened, and the child discovers that inside are stones, not candy. The box is closed again, and the experimenter now asks what another child, who has not looked inside the box, will think is inside. A child age 5 or older would probably reply that a naive child would think that the box contains candy. However, a much younger child is surprisingly likely to claim that the naive child would expect to find stones and, in fact, this child will deny that she *ever* expected to find anything else in the box! The difference can be understood in terms of developing theory of mind. Younger children do not understand how mental representations can be inconsistent with reality; for them, your beliefs about the world *must* be consistent with how things are. By contrast, 4- and 5-year-olds comprehend that reality can be represented in multiple ways and that people act on these mental representations, even though they may be incorrect (Wellman, 2002). Young children's dawning understanding of false belief is significant not only because it reveals an awareness of the independence of mental events from objective reality, but also because it is a gateway to the comprehension of other psychological realities, such as the privacy of personal mental experience, the creation of mistaken beliefs in others, and the mind's interpretive activity independent of experience. In short, young children begin to understand that how you feel or think need not be revealed, that others can be fooled, and that the mind operates independently of experience.

Understanding false belief, and other early achievements in developing theory of mind, emerges because young children are careful observers of other people and think insightfully about what they observe. As they watch people in goal-directed activity and see them express pleasure in their accomplishments and other emotions in different situations, and begin to overhear language incorporating mental state references (e.g., "I *thought* you were leaving . . . "), young children gradually construct an understanding of the mind. In addition, other social experiences are important catalysts for developing psychological understanding. In particular, young children's exposure to, and participation in, simple conversations with adults, siblings, and peers are a rich source of insight into mental events. In these conversations, children can learn about mental events through language that helps to make feelings and thoughts more explicit, they can compare their beliefs and expectations with those of others, and they can benefit from the insight provided by another into the psychological origins of the behavior of others whom they observe (Thompson, Laible, & Ontai, 2003). Thus, when parents discuss mental states (including emotions) more frequently and with greater elaborative detail, especially the causes of mental states in the child and others, preschoolers acquire a better understanding of people's thoughts, feelings, and intentions (Astington & Baird, 2005; Thompson et al., 2003). Indeed, some of the conceptual catalysts in social interaction to the development of theory of mind may arise surprisingly early, such as in the sensitivity of mothers to the psychological experiences of their infants (Meins et al., 2002).

More broadly, everyday conversations may also be important to children's acquisition of values, self-referent beliefs, causal assumptions, moral attributions, and other complex psychological inferences. Studies have shown, for example, that mothers' conversations about feelings contribute to early conscience development, and that disciplinary procedures requiring the child to reflect on the victim's feelings contribute to preschoolers' psychological understanding (Ruffman, Perner, & Parkin, 1999; Thompson et al., 2003). This may help to explain why individual differences in children's theory of mind understanding, particularly their comprehension of false belief and emotion understanding, are associated with children's social competence in friendship with peers (Denham et al., 2003; Dunn, Cutting, & Demetriou, 2000).

These remarkable advances in psychological understanding in early childhood set the stage for greater insight into people and the self. By ages 5 and 6, for example, young children begin to perceive others in terms of psychological motives and traits, and create expectations for others based on the traits they infer in them (Heyman & Gelman, 2000). They are also beginning to consider fairness in their peer relationships, particularly in relation to gender exclusion, although they have much to learn about social groups (Killen, Pisacane, Lee-Kim, & Ardile-Rey, 2001). Preschoolers are, in short, becoming more insightful in their psychological understanding of others, and these insights also extend to themselves.

There are important implications of these discoveries about developing psychological understanding for preschool mental health. Infants and young children clearly respond not only to people's behavior but also to the emotions, intentions, desires, and beliefs that they infer in others' actions and from what they learn about the psychological world from conversations with family members. Understanding the intergenerational influences that contribute to risk for internalizing and externalizing disorders in troubled families (e.g., inherited vulnerability, emotional climate of the home, coercive family interactions) must include the early sensitivity of young children to the intentions and emotions underlying their interactions with family members, and how attributional biases, moral judgments, and motivational evaluations are conveyed intergenerationally through parent–child conversation. Moreover, early peer relationships are also affected by developing psychological understanding; thus, the emotional vulnerability derived from interaction in a troubled family is likely to be manifested in young children's greater difficulty in peer sociability. Finally, although it is apparent that preschoolers are not sophisticated at misleading others concerning their thoughts and feelings, a rudimentary comprehension of the privacy of personal psychological experience is established in early achievements in theory of mind. This provides a foundation for psychological dissembling in the years that follow, together with a dawning awareness of how the mind itself constructs its own reality that can become enlisted for therapeutic purposes.

DEVELOPMENT OF SELF-UNDERSTANDING

Developing self-understanding in early childhood is important to mental health, because the self organizes experience and guides behavior. How young children represent themselves establishes continuity between an awareness of how one has been in the past and expectations for how one will be in the future. Developing autobiographical memory during the preschool years embeds self-understanding in representations of past events (Nelson & Fivush, 2004), and as children develop an awareness of their personal characteristics, it provides a guide to future action (Froming, Nasby, & McManus, 1998). For example, a young child's belief that she is shy may, when activated, discourage the child from interacting with a new child at school. Moreover, self-related beliefs can cause children to structure their experiences and environments in particular ways that influences the range of partners, challenges, and opportunities that children are likely to permit for themselves. Strong, coherent, and positive self-representations may offer a psychological buffer even in negative circumstances, whereas negative self-representations may be a risk factor for early clinical problems (Cicchetti & Rogosch, 1997; Harter, 1999). Both the development of a coherent, autonomous self and the specific characteristics of the developing self-concept have significant consequences for psychological development and risk of mental disorders.

Developmentally Emergent Features of the Self

Although the growth of an autonomous sense of self has traditionally been viewed as an accomplishment of childhood, many of the foundations of self-understanding emerge in infancy (Thompson, 2006). Early in the first year, for example, infants develop a prerepresentational form of self-awareness that derives from the perceptual experiences arising from their sensorimotor activity, affect, and experiences of agency in interaction with the world (Neisser, 1993). Young infants are highly attuned to the contingency between their own actions and the perceptual experiences that derive from them, and from this a nascent sense of "self" becomes constructed (Gergely & Watson, 1999). Later in the first year, the contingency of social interaction contributes to a dawning form of interpersonal or intersubjective self-awareness as infants strive to coordinate their own intentional, subjective states with those of others (e.g., in joint attention), and in their awareness that they can be the object of another's attention and affect. By age 18 months, another aspect of self-awareness emerges as toddlers become capable of featural self-recognition when identifying themselves in a mirror (Lewis & Brooks-Gunn, 1979), which heralds, to some researchers, the birth of the cognitive self-concept (Howe & Courage, 1997). These are each significant foundations to the gradual development of self-awareness and highlight that the emergence of the "self" is not a unitary process, but involves different facets of self-representation emerging at different periods in the early years.

It is not until around the second birthday that children's self-understanding begins to resemble the qualities of self that we recognize in older children. At this time, young children begin verbally self-referencing (e.g., "Me, too!"), as well as asserting their competence (e.g., by refusing assistance) and describing their experiences using internal state words, such as references to feelings and desires (Bretherton & Beeghly, 1982; Stipek, Gralinski, & Kopp, 1990). Young children are also sensitive to how others evaluate them, partly because they are beginning to conceptualize and apply standards of conduct to their own behavior; thus, others' evaluations of them are important and influential (Stipek, Recchia, & McClintic, 1992; Thompson, Meyer, & McGinley, 2006). This contributes to the earliest experiences of self-referential emotions, such as pride, shame, guilt, or embarrassment, that expand emotional experience and link the development of emotion and self (Lewis, 2000; Stipek et al., 1992).

By the third year, therefore, self-representations have become globally affective and evaluative in nature. Moreover, in contrast with the traditional view that young children perceive themselves exclusively in terms of physical appearance and behavior (e.g., brown hair, runs fast), there is growing evidence that even young children develop a coherent, psychologically oriented self-concept by 3½ to 4 years of age. This becomes apparent when researchers, rather than asking children to describe themselves using open-ended questions (which tend to elicit concrete self-descriptors), instead invite children to describe their characteristics by choosing from contrasting pairs of descriptive attributes (e.g., "I like to be with other people" vs. "I like to be by myself") (e.g., Brown, Mangelsdorf, Agathen, & Ho, 2004; Eder, 1990; Marsh, Ellis, & Craven, 2002; Measelle, Ablow, Cowan, & Cowan, 1998). Studies using such measures show that young children are capable of representing their psychological and emotional qualities in conceptually coherent ways, describing individual differences in their physical skills, academic capabilities, relationships with parents and peers, social competence, and even self-characterizations of feelings relevant to depression, anxiety, and aggression or hostility. Moreover, young children's self-descriptions show stability over time and are consistent with mothers' and teachers' reports of children's personality characteristics (Brown et al., 2004; Eder & Mangelsdorf, 1997; Measelle et al., 1998).

In summary, although further research is needed to elucidate the meaning inherent in young children's use of trait labels (which probably lack the rich meaning inherent in how older people use these concepts), and there is considerable growth yet to occur in their self-awareness, it seems apparent that children are thinking of themselves in psychologically relevant ways from late in the preschool years. This raises at least two important considerations for preschool mental health. First, it suggests that a psychological self-concept emerges surprisingly early and is thus likely to be significantly affected by the family emotional climate in early childhood, as discussed below. Second, because psychological self-awareness is slowly emerging in the early years, child clinicians must be cautious in their inferences from preschoolers' statements about themselves by remembering that young children often have different underlying conceptions in their use of trait labels than do adults (see Luby & Belden, Chapter 10, this volume, on mood disorders). A young child who proclaims that she can accomplish impossible feats or does not like to be with other people may not be reflecting the same self-attributions that would be true if these statements were from an older child or adult.

By the end of the preschool years, therefore, young children's self-understanding provides a foundation for how they will see themselves in the years to come, although there remains significant growth in the depth, complexity, and nuance of self-understanding to come. Even so, by age 5, children perceive themselves in psychologically complex ways, evaluate their characteristics and accomplishments (with contributions from others' evaluations of them), and experience a range of self-referential emotions. Moreover, children of this age can also regard themselves within a broad temporal framework—relating their past experiences to future expectations—that constitutes a conceptual foundation for autobiographical memory (Nelson & Fivush, 2004; Povinelli, 2001). These accomplishments also contribute to the significant advances in self-regulation that occur during the preschool years, with children becoming more capable of managing their behavior, attention, thinking, and emotions than was true in infancy, although important advances are yet to come (Fox & Calkins, 2003; Kopp, 1982). The preschooler has become a psychologically complex individual in his or her own eyes, as well as in the eyes of others.

One implication is that early childhood influences have important consequences for developing psychological self-understanding, and that self-concept might receive clinical attention in evaluation of young children at psychological risk for mood disorders and other difficulties. There is evidence, for example, that aversive early caregiving experiences can profoundly affect many features of developing self-representation in early childhood. Maltreated toddlers and young children exhibit more negative or neutral affect in visual self-recognition, for example, and less frequently use verbal self-reference and internal state words (particularly negative emotion words) compared with nonmaltreated children (Beeghly & Cicchetti, 1994; Schneider-Rosen & Cicchetti, 1991). Moreover, consistent with their sensitivity to others' evaluations of themselves, young children are not only prone to negative self-evaluations when caregivers likewise appraise their performance, but these negative self-assessments may also, in some circumstances, contribute to risk for later depressive disorders (Kistner, Ziegert, Castro, & Robertson, 2001). The findings of studies such as these underscore the associations between caregiving relationships, the development of self-understanding, risk for psychopathology, and manifestations of clinical disorders arising in early childhood.

Influences on Developing Self-Representations

Early relational experience is important to developing self-understanding in several ways. As earlier noted, caregivers and others who matter to the child contribute a valuational dimension to self-understanding, arising from how they regard the child and how it is expressed, from the affect with which they view the child's mirror image to how they evaluate the child's accomplishments, misbehavior, and characteristics. In light of the importance of these